POCKET GUIDE

CRITICAL CARE PLACEMENTS

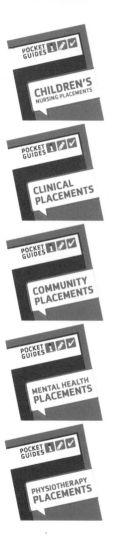

Pocket Guides

"A very useful, well-written and practical pocket book for any level of student nurse preparing for clinical placement. This book is also a great resource for lecturers and mentors to have, to help students get the most out of their placement time." ★★★★★

"This is such a useful guide that has just the right amount of need to know info for student nurses on clinical placement, as well as loads of little tips scattered throughout. A must-have for student nurses on placements!" ★★★★★

"Full of everything you need to know as a student nurse on placement. Written by students for students. Helpful little references to help with abbreviations and common medications. A must for any student about to head on placement." ★★★★★

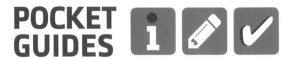

POCKET GUIDES

CRITICAL CARE PLACEMENTS

Rachel Dodd and Rachel Parkinson
Edited by Ruth Magowan

Queen Margaret University
Edinburgh

Lantern

ISBN: 9781908625816
First published in 2020 by Lantern Publishing Ltd

Lantern Publishing Limited, The Old Hayloft, Vantage
Business Park, Bloxham Road, Banbury OX16 9UX, UK
www.lanternpublishing.com

British Library Cataloguing in Publication Data
A catalogue record for this book is available from the British Library

The authors and publisher have made every attempt to ensure
the content of this book is up to date and accurate. However,
healthcare knowledge and information is changing all the time
so the reader is advised to double-check any information in
this text on drug usage, treatment procedures, the use of
equipment, etc. to confirm that it complies with the latest safety
recommendations, standards of practice and legislation, as well as
local Trust policies and procedures. Students are advised to check
with their tutor and/or practice supervisor before carrying out
any of the procedures in this textbook.

Typeset by Medlar Publishing Solutions Pvt Ltd, India
Printed and bound in the UK

Last digit is the print number: 10 9 8 7 6 5 4 3 2 1

Personal information

Name:. . . . .

Mobile:. . . . .

Address during placement:. . . . .

UNIVERSITY DETAILS

University:. . . . .

Programme leader:. . . . .

Personal tutor:. . . . .

PLACEMENT DETAILS

Placement area:. . . . .

Practice Education Facilitator:. . . . .

Link lecturer:. . . . .

CONTACT IN CASE OF EMERGENCY

Name:. . . . .

Contact number (mobile):. . . . .

Contact number (home/work):. . . . .

Contents

Resources

Foreword

I am delighted to endorse this pocket guide written *for* student nurses *by* student nurses. Rachel Dodd and Rachel Parkinson have been passionate about this project – their desire to pass information on to fellow nursing students that they wish they had had when in intensive and critical care areas. These areas of care can undoubtedly be daunting for any nurse and this book gives accessible and clear information about common illnesses and procedures that students are likely to encounter. Critical care placements provide a diversity of experience and a huge amount of new information. This book provides the essentials that you need to know.

The authors have collaborated in their writing and reviewing team with specialists from practice, academics and current students to ensure that the information in the book is current and relevant. It has been my privilege to support the writing of this book, and I look forward to continuing to work with the authors and wider team of collaborators in their ongoing work to extend the knowledge base and application of person-centred care to critical care and practice. I wish the team every success in all their future endeavours.

Ruth E. Magowan

BA (Hons) Nursing, MSc, PGCE, RSCN, RGN, SFHEA

Senior Lecturer, Nursing Division, School of Health Sciences, Queen Margaret University, Edinburgh

Clinical Nurse Specialist, Borders General Hospital

Preface

This handbook is primarily written for student nurses. Critical care placements provide a diversity of experience and a huge amount of new information. At the time of writing this book we were both nursing students in our third year. We had just completed our critical care placements and were discussing how difficult it was to take in the huge amount of information each day. We decided to write this book to help other students understand the complex area that is critical care.

The absolute best advice we can offer is simply to get involved. This book will detail a variety of roles of healthcare professionals during specific treatments, including your role as a student nurse. We know that some situations can seem daunting and if you do not want to be hands-on immediately, that is OK; however, you can gain so much from simply observing, so never just walk away from a new experience.

Ask questions, research information that is new to you – if you are ever unsure if you should pull the emergency buzzer, pull it, watch everything and get involved in as much as you can, and you will get the most out of your placement.

All the information used in this handbook has been sourced from published evidence. We have included a reading list in *Chapter 21* if you wish to read further into a specific area. The list is compiled from information that we found easy to understand and is accessible for everyone.

Rachel Dodd and Rachel Parkinson
Queen Margaret University

Acknowledgements

Creating this handbook has not been without its struggles. There have been many people who have guided us during the writing process, to ensure it is as useful and as practical as possible. We would like to thank Professor Brendan McCormack for reviewing and discussing with us the person-centred elements; Ronnie Dornan for evaluating and assisting with the physiological aspects; Stephanie Norton-Alexander for giving us the perspective from another nursing student; and all of the students who participated in our survey and took the time to listen and discuss our ideas with us. The biggest thank you must go to Ruth Magowan, for without her, there would simply be no book. Ruth's guidance and advice have been invaluable throughout this process.

The publishers would like to thank Kirstie Paterson and Jessica Wallar, authors of *Clinical Placements*, the first in the Pocket Guide series, and Kath MacDonald, their editor, for permission to use some of the content from their book as well as the overall framework.

Abbreviations

ABG	arterial blood gas
ACS	acute coronary syndrome
AED	automated external defibrillator
ATLS	Advanced Trauma Life Support
AVPU	alert, voice, pain, unresponsive
BP	blood pressure
bpm	beats per minute
COPD	chronic obstructive pulmonary disorder
CRT	capillary refill time
ECG	electrocardiogram
GCS	Glasgow Coma Scale
GTN	glyceryl trinitrate
IV	intravenous
JVP	jugular venous pulse
MAP	mean arterial pressure
MI	myocardial infarction
NEWS	National Early Warning Score
NG	nasogastric
O_2	oxygen
PCC	person-centred care
PCI	percutaneous coronary intervention
PEA	pulseless electrical activity
PR	per rectum
PV	per vagina
SBAR	situation, background, assessment, recommendation
TIA	transient ischaemic attack
UTI	urinary tract infection
VF	ventricular fibrillation
VT	ventricular tachycardia

> Confusion in the use of abbreviations has been cited as the reason for some clinical incidents. Therefore you should use these abbreviations with caution and only in line with local Trusts' Clinical Governance recommendations which vary between departments!

Introduction

This handbook has been designed so that nursing students have quick access to relevant, condensed and understandable information when on placement in a critical care area. As you have already experienced a clinical placement, you will have an idea of the fundamentals of nursing practice. This book will help you to further develop your practice by expanding your knowledge and skill set in a critical care setting.

The first part of the book focuses on Advanced Life Support and assessments that can be used when a new patient arrives into your care or when someone deteriorates.

The second part of the book contains explanations of conditions you are likely to see and has information on definitions, signs and symptoms, assessment and possible treatment plans.

The third part of the book is a toolkit that has advice on how to carry out physical tasks in a critical care area. Parts of the toolkit have deliberately been designed for patient participation. This is to encourage collaboration, inclusion and participation between patients and students.

There is also some space in the book to note down your own thoughts and anything else you find relevant. We hope you find this book to be helpful in your critical care placement.

 Notes

Person-centred care

Person-centred care (PCC) is a term that will be used throughout your placement. It means ensuring that your patient is at the centre of their care, including them in decisions and enabling them to be a proactive member of the team. As a student nurse you are in a unique position, in that you do not necessarily have the same responsibilities and pressures that staff members have. Try to take the time to talk to the people you are caring for and learn about the things in their life that matter to them. Care for your patients according to their beliefs and values – so it is important to find out what these are from the patients themselves or from a family member if they aren't in a position to communicate these with you.

A model that might help you think about PCC is the Person-centred Practice Framework (McCormack and McCance, 2017) shown on the next page. This model has the person requiring care at the centre and is framed by the person-centred processes (the petals on the flower) and surrounded by the organisational systems and prerequisites of the practitioner that are required for working in a person-centred way.

✎ Notes

_____

_____

_____

_____

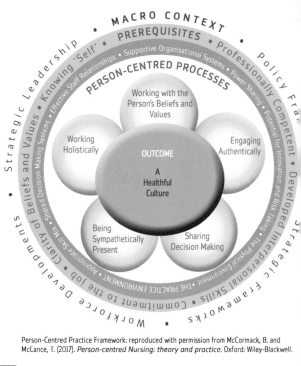

Person-Centred Practice Framework: reproduced with permission from McCormack, B. and McCance, T. (2017). *Person-centred Nursing: theory and practice*. Oxford: Wiley-Blackwell.

Notes

As a student nurse you may feel that within critical care areas it can be harder to implement person-centred care. However, person-centred care transcends all areas of practice, and we would suggest that this approach is essential in critical care. It is often the simple things such as taking the time to know a person's name, doing what you can to find out the person's values and beliefs or advocating for the patient's wants and needs, that demonstrate person-centred care. Using person-centred ways of working is not something that takes a lot of time, but it makes a big difference to the people you care for.

Notes

Notes

Advanced Life Support and assessments

3.1 Cardiac arrest definition

Working in critical care areas can be daunting, as your patients are seriously unwell. They can deteriorate quickly and as a student nurse you may witness a cardiac arrest. A cardiorespiratory arrest can be defined as the sudden cessation of the heartbeat and cardiac function, resulting in failure of effective circulation and respiration.

ℹ Cardiac arrest

A cardiac arrest is identified by:

- loss of consciousness
- absence of central pulse (carotid/femoral)
- absence of spontaneous respiration.

3.2 Basic Life Support

It is important to remember that within critical care areas most cardiac arrests are anticipated. Therefore, it is important to recognise cardiac arrest, summon help and commence Basic Life Support as seen in the algorithm below.

✎ Notes

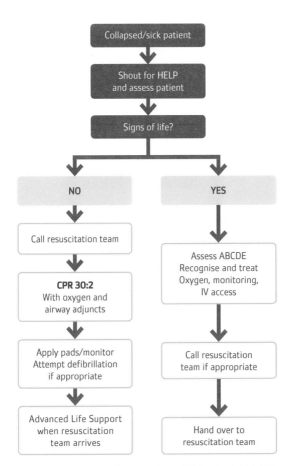

Collapsed/sick patient

↓

Shout for HELP
and assess patient

↓

Signs of life?

NO

↓

Call resuscitation team

↓

CPR 30:2
With oxygen and
airway adjuncts

↓

Apply pads/monitor
Attempt defibrillation
if appropriate

↓

Advanced Life Support
when resuscitation
team arrives

YES

↓

Assess ABCDE
Recognise and treat
Oxygen, monitoring,
IV access

↓

Call resuscitation
team if appropriate

↓

Hand over to
resuscitation team

In-hospital cardiac arrest algorithm (Resuscitation Council, 2015). Reproduced with the kind permission of the Resuscitation Council (UK).

3.3 Management of cardiac arrest

The management of cardiac arrests has been standardised by the Advanced Life Support (ALS) protocols developed by the Resuscitation Council (UK)(2015), as seen below. However, it is still important to familiarise yourself with local policy where you are on placement. VF (ventricular fibrillation) and VT (ventricular tachycardia) are the only shockable rhythms (see *Chapter 15* for more information on shockable and non-shockable rhythms). The optimum treatment for VF and pulseless VT is early defibrillation (see *Section 3.4*).

✎ Notes

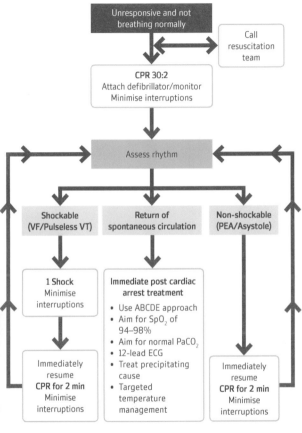

```
Unresponsive and not
breathing normally
                              Call resuscitation
                              team

CPR 30:2
Attach defibrillator/monitor
Minimise interruptions

            Assess rhythm

Shockable          Return of            Non-shockable
(VF/Pulseless VT)  spontaneous          (PEA/Asystole)
                   circulation

1 Shock            Immediate post cardiac   Immediately
Minimise           arrest treatment         resume
interruptions                               CPR for 2 min
                   • Use ABCDE approach     Minimise
                   • Aim for SpO₂ of        interruptions
                     94–98%
Immediately        • Aim for normal PaCO₂
resume             • 12-lead ECG
CPR for 2 min      • Treat precipitating
Minimise             cause
interruptions      • Targeted
                     temperature
                     management
```

Unresponsive and not breathing normally

Call resuscitation team

CPR 30:2
Attach defibrillator/monitor
Minimise interruptions

Assess rhythm

Shockable (VF/Pulseless VT)

Return of spontaneous circulation

Non-shockable (PEA/Asystole)

1 Shock
Minimise interruptions

Immediate post cardiac arrest treatment
- Use ABCDE approach
- Aim for SpO_2 of 94–98%
- Aim for normal $PaCO_2$
- 12-lead ECG
- Treat precipitating cause
- Targeted temperature management

Immediately resume **CPR for 2 min** Minimise interruptions

Immediately resume **CPR for 2 min** Minimise interruptions

(continued)

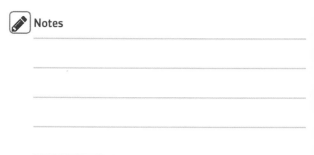

During CPR	Treat Reversible Causes	Consider
• Ensure high quality chest compressions • Minimise interruptions to compressions • Give oxygen • Use waveform capnography • Continuous compressions when advanced airway in place • Vascular access (intravenous or intraosseous) • Give adrenaline every 3–5 min • Give amiodarone after 3 shocks	• Hypoxia • Hypovolaemia • Hypo-/ hyperkalaemia/ metabolic • Hypothermia • Thrombosis – coronary or pulmonary • Tension pneumothorax • Tamponade – cardiac • Toxins	• Ultrasound imaging • Mechanical chest compressions to facilitate transfer/ treatment • Coronary angiography and percutaneous coronary intervention • Extracorporeal CPR

Adult advanced life support algorithm (Resuscitation Council, 2015). Reproduced with the kind permission of the Resuscitation Council (UK).

✏️ **Notes**

_____

_____

_____

_____

_____

3.4 Correct placement of defibrillation pads

If a defibrillator (also known as an AED; automated external defibrillator) is used when you are on shift, go and watch and, if possible, get involved. You may be asked to place the defib pads on the patient.

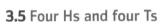

3.5 Four Hs and four Ts

The 4 Hs and 4 Ts is a mnemonic used to help remember the reversible causes of cardiac arrest. To successfully resuscitate you must reverse the cause.

The 4 Hs		
Hypoxia (low O_2)	→	Give O_2
Hypovolaemia (low blood volume)	→	Give blood products and do blood tests
Hypothermia (low temperature)	→	Take core temperature and warm slowly
Hypercalcaemia (imbalance of ions)	→	Blood tests and give ion that is missing
The 4 Ts		
Thrombolytic disorders (e.g. MI)	→	Give clot-busting medication; CPR will help move clot
Toxins (anaphylaxis or overdose)	→	Blood test and toxicology
Tamponade (blood in pericardial space)	→	Blood has to be removed
Tension pneumothorax (collapsed lung)	→	Chest tube

3.6 Effective CPR

Ensure high quality chest compressions:

- Depth of 5–6 cm
- Rate of 100–120 compressions per minute
- Allow the chest to recoil completely after each compression
- Take approximately the same amount of time for compression and relaxation
- Minimise any interruptions to chest compression (hands-off time).

Always remember the ABCDE. You cannot move on to the next step until the previous one has been resolved. For example, you cannot start trying to treat breathing issues without a secure airway. Further information about ABCDE can be found in *Section 4.1*.

A	Airway
B	Breathing
C	Circulation
D	Disability
E	Exposure

When working in Critical Care areas you may witness and be asked to participate in a resuscitation attempt. Unlike in movies and TV shows, these are usually anticipated and very well organised. A doctor or an experienced nurse will take charge and allocate roles. Communication between the members of the multidisciplinary group is key to a smooth and effective resuscitation attempt. The doctor in charge will usually look after the airway, someone will start chest compressions and there will be someone to take over once they get tired. While someone starts compressions the resus trolley will be brought, and defibrillation pads will be placed on the chest with minimal interruption to compressions. Another person will be responsible for drawing up and administering the drugs that are required, while someone will record the rounds of CPR and the medications given. As a student you may be asked to do compressions or help draw up medications with another nurse.

Further information can be found on the Resuscitation Council (UK) website, www.resus.org.uk

> Also consider looking after yourself:
>
> As a nursing student you see a lot of hard things to deal with emotionally. It is important to reflect and debrief about the situations you are involved in within your practice. It's good to seek out support from others if required, to help deal with what you may witness on placement. Person-centred care is not just the care of others around you, but also includes self-care.

Notes

_____

_____

_____

_____

_____

Resuscitation Council (2015) *Resuscitation Guidelines*. Available at: bit.ly/Resus-2015

Nurses continuously assess the people they are caring for. It is important to remember that an assessment does not need to follow a particular framework to be classed as an assessment, and your eyes are one of the most helpful tools when assessing patients.

The first assessment that should be carried out when a patient arrives in a critical care area, or when a patient quickly deteriorates, is the ABCDE assessment. The below assessments are usually carried out by the entire team upon arrival; however, nurses may work through these independently upon discovering a deteriorating patient. Remember to shout for help if needed.

4.1 ABCDE assessment

A	Airway
B	Breathing
C	Circulation
D	Disability
E	Exposure

✐ Notes

_____

_____

_____

_____

A – Airway

Airway obstruction is an emergency. Airway obstructions can cause hypoxia. Seek help immediately.

Signs of airway obstruction:

- Seesaw breathing
- Use of accessory muscles
- Cyanosis.

Treatment of airway obstruction:

When breathing without difficulty, the chest and abdomen rise and fall together. During seesaw breathing, the abdomen and chest move opposite to one another. On inhalation the abdomen will fall and the chest will rise, whereas during exhalation the abdomen will rise and the chest will fall.

1. Open the airway:
   - Head tilt chin lift or jaw thrust may open the airway
   - Airway suctioning to clear secretions
   - Insert an oropharyngeal or nasopharyngeal airway
   - The patient should be intubated if the above fails to clear the obstruction.
2. Give oxygen at high concentration:
   - Give high flow oxygen using a mask with an oxygen reservoir. Ensure that the oxygen flow is sufficient (usually 15 L/min).

B – Breathing

Conditions such as tension pneumothorax, acute severe asthma and pulmonary oedema should be diagnosed and treated here.

Look, listen and feel for signs of respiratory distress including sweating, cyanosis, the use of accessory muscles and abdominal breathing.

- Count the respiratory rate. A high (>25/min) or increasing respiratory rate is an indicator that the patient may deteriorate suddenly.
- Assess the depth of each breath, the pattern of breathing and observe if the chest expansion is equal on both sides.
- Note any chest deformity.
- Look for a raised jugular venous pulse (JVP; see figure below), especially in acute severe asthma or a tension pneumothorax.

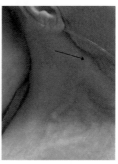

Raised JVP. Reproduced under a CC-BY-SA-3.0 licence. Attribution: James Heilman, MD.

- Observe any chest drains that may be present, particularly the volume and patency of drains.
- Remember that if the abdomen is distended it may limit diaphragmatic movement, thereby worsening respiratory distress.
- Record the SpO_2 reading. (Remember that if the patient is receiving supplemental oxygen the SpO_2 reading may be normal despite a high $PaCo_2$.)
- Listen to the patient's breath sounds: rattling noises indicate the presence of secretions. Stridor, or wheeze, suggests partial, but significant airway obstruction.
- Percuss the chest: hyper-resonance suggests a pneumothorax. Dullness usually indicates consolidation or pleural fluid.

- Auscultate the chest: bronchial breathing indicates lung consolidation. Absent or reduced sounds suggest a pneumothorax, pleural fluid or lung consolidation caused by complete obstruction.
- Treat the cause.
- All patients should be treated with high flow oxygen; however, be wary of CO_2-retaining patients (COPD).
- If the patient's depth or rate of breathing is insufficient, or absent, use bag-mask or pocket mask ventilation.

> If possible, stand at the bottom of the bed when assessing if the patient's chest is expanding equally, as it is easier to see from this angle.

C – Circulation

It should be assumed that hypovolaemia is the primary cause of shock until proven otherwise, in both medical and surgical emergencies.

Patients with cool peripheries and tachycardia should be given IV fluids, unless there are obvious signs of a cardiac cause.

Pay attention to the hands and digits: are they blue, pink, pale or mottled?

- Assess the limb temperature and colour by feeling the patient's hands: are they cool or warm?
- Measure the capillary refill time (CRT). Apply pressure for 5 seconds on a fingertip held at heart level (or just above) with enough pressure to cause skin blanching. The normal CRT is usually <2 seconds. A prolonged CRT suggests poor peripheral perfusion. Other factors such as cold surroundings, poor lighting and old age can prolong CRT.
- Assess the veins: when hypovolaemia is present, they may be underfilled or collapsed.

- Count the patient's pulse rate (or preferably heart rate by listening to the heart with a stethoscope).
- Palpate pulses: feel for presence of pulse, rate, quality, regularity and equality.

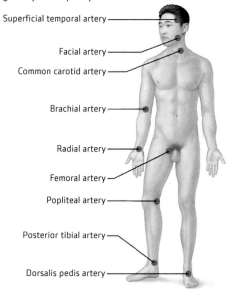

Superficial temporal artery

Facial artery

Common carotid artery

Brachial artery

Radial artery

Femoral artery

Popliteal artery

Posterior tibial artery

Dorsalis pedis artery

Pulse points over major arteries.

Barely palpable central pulses suggest a poor cardiac output, whilst a bounding pulse may indicate sepsis.

Measure the patient's blood pressure (BP). Remember in shock, BP may be normal, because the body is compensating.

- Auscultate the heart. Listen for a murmur – can you clearly make out the sounds and does the audible heart rate correspond to the pulse rate?

- Look for other signs of a poor cardiac output:
  - reduced conscious level
  - oliguria (urine volume <0.5 ml/kg/h)
- Look *under the bed covers* for external haemorrhage from wounds or drains or evidence of concealed haemorrhage.
- Treat the cause.
- Treatment should aim to replace lost fluid, control haemorrhage and restore tissue perfusion.
- Insert one or more large intravenous cannulas. Short, wide-bore cannulas should be placed, as they enable the highest flow.
- Take blood from the cannula for investigations and cross-matching, before giving intravenous fluid.
- A bolus of 500 ml of warmed crystalloid solution (e.g. Hartmann's solution) should be given over no more than 15 min if the patient is hypotensive.
- Reassess the heart rate and BP regularly, aiming for the patient's normal BP or, if this is unknown, a target >100 mmHg systolic.
- If the patient does not improve, repeat the fluid challenge.
- Look for symptoms and signs of cardiac failure:
  - dyspnoea
  - increased heart rate
  - raised JVP
  - a third heart sound and pulmonary crackles on auscultation.

If these symptoms occur decrease the fluid infusion rate or stop the fluids altogether. Alternative means of improving tissue perfusion should be used (inotropes or vasopressors).

1. If the patient has chest pain and suspected ACS (acute coronary syndrome), record a 12-lead ECG early.
2. Immediate general treatment for ACS:
   - aspirin 300 mg, orally, crushed or chewed
   - nitroglycerine, as sublingual glyceryl trinitrate (GTN) (tablet or spray).

- oxygen – only give oxygen if the patient's SpO$_2$ is <94% breathing air alone.
- morphine (or diamorphine).

D – Disability

Common causes of unconsciousness include hypoxia, hypercapnia, cerebral hypoperfusion or recent administration of sedative or analgesic drugs.

- Review and treat the ABCs – hypoxia and hypotension should be treated or ruled out.
- Check the patient's Kardex for reversible drug-induced causes of depressed consciousness. Give the reversing agent when possible.
- Examine the pupils, looking at size, equality and reaction to light.
- Assess conscious level using Glasgow Coma Scale (see *Section 12.1*) or AVPU:

A	**Alert**	Patient is alert
V	**Voice**	Patient responds to voice
P	**Pain**	Patient responds to pain
U	**Unresponsive**	Patient is unresponsive

- Exclude hypoglycaemia using finger prick test. In a patient who is just about to, or has just arrested, use a venous or arterial blood sample, as finger prick samples can be unreliable in very sick patients. Blood glucose should be remeasured to monitor efficiency of treatment.
- Remember to document AVPU, GCS and blood sugar on NEWS chart and escalate as appropriate.

E – Exposure

- To carry out a complete examination of the body, the patient may need to be fully exposed. The patient's dignity should be upheld at all times. Heat loss should be minimised as much as possible.

4.2 Trauma assessment

The advanced trauma life support (ATLS) guidelines derive from the Resuscitation Council UK chain of survival. ATLS contains two different assessments, both of which should be used.

Primary survey

This survey has been adapted from the ABCDE assessment above and is designed to quickly find life-threatening issues and address these as they are discovered.

Ac – Airway with cervical spine

- Obtain an airway.
- Cervical spinal injury should be assumed when a patient has suffered significant blunt force trauma or professionals believe an injury has occurred above the clavicles, and should only be ruled out after definitive testing.
- To prevent further injury to the spinal cord, the neck should be immobilised using a rigid cervical collar and head blocks with tape.

> Remember to position yourself carefully so that the patient can see you when you are talking to them, as they cannot turn with the collar in place.

B – Breathing

- Count the respiratory rate
- Evaluate breathing
- Record SpO$_2$

- Pay attention to drains
- Treat the cause of respiratory distress (remember that emotions and mental health can be a cause of physical symptoms).

C – Circulation and control of haemorrhage

- If a catastrophic bleed occurs this may take precedence over breathing.
- Treatment of catastrophic haemorrhage:
    - direct pressure
    - elevation
    - tourniquet.

If a patient is hypotensive this should be assumed to be caused by haemorrhage until proven otherwise.

- If a patient is tachycardic but has a normal BP, hypovolaemia should be suspected.
- Anxiety, confusion and agitation can alert professionals to decreased cellular perfusion. Nurses may spot this first as they will be communicating with the patient.
- Large bore cannulas should be inserted.
- Initiate a fluid challenge. Aim for a systolic BP of above 70 mmHg.
    - 2 L of warmed Hartmann's solution should be given initially.
    - 250 ml boluses are then given if no sufficient response.
- Blood should be replaced.
- A blood sample should be obtained.
- Place a 12-lead ECG.
- A nasogastric (NG) tube should be considered to decompress the stomach.

Dolan, B. and Holt, L. (2013) *Accident and Emergency: theory and practice*, 3rd edition. Elsevier Health Sciences.

- A catheter should then be placed to record urine output; aim for >0.5 ml per hour, per kg.
- Fluid chart should be started.

D – Disability

- Review and treat the ABCs: hypoxia and hypotension should be treated or ruled out.
- Check the patient's Kardex for reversible drug-induced consciousness. Give the reversing agent when possible.
- Examine the pupils, looking at size, equality and reaction to light.
- Assess conscious level using Glasgow Coma Scale or AVPU.
- Exclude hypoglycaemia.

E – Exposure

- Patient's clothing should be removed to check for further injuries; the patient should then be re-dressed as appropriate.
- Patient should be carefully log-rolled to examine the back.

F – Fahrenheit (control of environment)

- Trauma patients are at a higher risk of suffering from hypothermia as their bodies are more likely to have been exposed to cold and wet conditions. Severe blood loss can also lower the body's core temperature.
- Hypothermia can be prevented by:
  - warmed blankets
  - warmed IV fluids
  - reduced exposure of patient.

Top tip

Remember that C (Circulation and control of haemorrhage) may come before A (Airway with cervical spine) in this survey as a catastrophic haemorrhage can result in immediate death.

Secondary survey

The second part of the survey is a complete head-to-toe evaluation of the patient. The purpose of this survey is to identify injuries that the patient has sustained. Each area of the body should be examined to rule out injury.

Below is a mnemonic to help remember every area that should be checked. Remember that it is important to respect the patient's dignity at all times.

Mnemonic	Secondary survey
Has	Head/skull
My	Maxillofacial
Critical	Cervical spine
Care	Chest
Assessed	Abdomen
Patient's	Pelvis
Priorities	Perineum
Or	Orifices (PR/PV)
Next	Neurological
Management	Musculoskeletal
Decision?	Diagnostic tests / definitive care

Resuscitation Council (2019) *The ABCDE Approach*. Available at: bit.ly/RC-ABCDE

Hughes, S. (2006) ATLS secondary survey mnemonic: Has My Critical Care Assessed Patient's Priorities Or Next Management Decision? *Emergency Medical Journal*, **23**: 661–662.

Common conditions in critical care

Shock is a complex clinical syndrome characterised by a lack of adequate tissue and organ perfusion to such an extent that the oxygen and nutritional needs of the cells are not being met. This results in the body's cells and organs being unable to function adequately. Failure to treat will lead to multiorgan failure. In order to treat shock, you must treat the cause.

5.1 Types of shock

Shock is classified according to cause. There are three distinct mechanisms that may lead to hypoperfusion of the tissues.

- Hypovolaemia – there is not enough blood to carry oxygen and nutrients around the body
- Pump failure (cardiogenic) – the heart is unable to pump the blood around the body effectively
- Distributive – occurs when there is a distribution problem within the body. Blood volume and cardiac output are adequate but widespread vasoconstriction leads to pooling of blood and reduces venous return to the heart. Neurogenic, septic and anaphylactic shock are forms of distributive shock.

Hypovolaemic shock

The causes of hypovolaemic shock are:

- loss of blood through haemorrhage
- loss of plasma (e.g. severe burns)
- loss of bodily fluids through diarrhoea, vomiting or sweating
- failure to drink sufficient fluids.

Cardiogenic shock

Events which reduce the ability of the heart to pump efficiently result in cardiogenic shock; these include:

- myocardial infarction
- cardiac arrhythmias
- disorders of the lungs (e.g. tension pneumothorax or pulmonary emboli).

Distributive shock

In this form of shock cardiac output and blood volume are adequate; however, widespread vasoconstriction leads to pooling of blood and causes a reduction in venous return to the heart. Within this category of shock are neurogenic, septic and anaphylactic shock.

Neurogenic shock

In neurogenic shock, sympathetic and parasympathetic nervous control is lost. The venous 'tone' responsible for maintaining normal BP and venous return is lost, and blood pools in the venules and capillaries. Common causes include:

- severe head injury
- spinal injury
- drug reaction and anaesthetics
- neurological illness (e.g. Guillain–Barré syndrome).

Septic shock

Damage is caused by an overwhelming bacterial infection. The bacteria cause damage by releasing endotoxins that cause vasodilation and increased capillary permeability. Fluid leaks out of the capillaries, causing hypotension and ultimately hypovolaemia. More information can be found on sepsis in *Chapter 6*.

Anaphylactic shock

Anaphylaxis occurs as a result of an antigen–antibody response in sensitive individuals. Antigens combine with immunoglobulin E antibodies on the surface of mast cells throughout the body and these cells degranulate, releasing histamine and prostaglandins into the circulation. The release of these into the circulation causes the capillaries to become more permeable and results in widespread oedema, which can rapidly cause death if not treated with adrenaline. Antigens can be introduced through ingestion, injection or inhalation.

5.2 Stages of shock

Whatever the initial cause of the shock response, the pathophysiological response remains the same. The inadequate perfusion of the organs deprives the cells of oxygen, resulting in cell damage.

Shock occurs in stages:

Compensatory stage

In the initial stage of shock, the body is able to compensate for the changes that are occurring at a cellular level due to homeostatic mechanisms. The body is trying to preserve blood flow to the vital organs by the vasoconstriction of blood vessels and increasing the heart rate.

 Signs and symptoms that someone is in compensatory shock:

- Rapid, weak pulse
- Skin becomes cold as blood is diverted from the peripheries
- Deep rapid breathing
- They may become confused and disorientated as blood supply to the brain is reduced.

Progressive stage

Failing to treat the cause of shock means that the person will move on from the compensatory shock. The body's homeostatic mechanisms are unable to compensate and begin to fail. Cells throughout the body begin to malfunction.

Signs and symptoms that someone is in the progressive stage of shock:

- Hyperventilation caused by metabolic acidosis
- Reduced blood flow to the brain causes a reduced level of consciousness
- Reduced blood volume and flow results in poor renal perfusion, which results in reduced urine output
- The liver is no longer able to conjugate bilirubin and jaundice occurs
- The heart's ability to pump blood is so reduced that it is unable even to supply the needs of the cardiac muscle, and becomes weaker and weaker.

Irreversible stage

Early intervention can mean that homeostasis can be restored, but once cell breakdown and acidosis reach a critical level, the damage is irreversible and death will follow despite all interventions.

 Notes

_____

_____

_____

_____

31

Sepsis is a life-threatening condition that occurs when the body has an abnormal overreaction to an infection. This can result in organ dysfunction, tissue damage and death.

6.1 Signs and symptoms of sepsis

Signs and symptoms can vary from patient to patient. Not all signs and symptoms need to be present for sepsis to be diagnosed.

- Hypotension (systolic BP <90 mmHg)
- Temperature (<36.0°C or >38.3°C)
- Lowered oxygen saturation (<94%)
- Decreased urine output (<0.5 ml/kg)
- Pulse >90
- Resp. rate >20
- Decreased CRT (>2 seconds)
- White blood cells (<4.0 x 10^9/L or >12.0 x 10^9/L)
- High level of creatinine in blood (creatinine levels will vary depending on age and gender)
- High lactate level in blood (>2 mmol/L)
- Decreased level of consciousness
- The person may feel cool and clammy to touch
- The person may feel extremely unwell.

Remember TIME!

Temperature – is it higher or lower than normal?
Infection – are there any signs or symptoms of infection?
Mental decline – is the person confused, sleepy or difficult to rouse?
Extremely ill – are they in severe pain or discomfort?

6.2 Treatment of sepsis

Treatment should be started **as quickly as possible** when sepsis is suspected or diagnosed. Nurses have a key role in helping to identify sepsis. If you suspect someone you are caring for may have sepsis, discuss this with your practice supervisor as soon as possible.

1. **Ensure a senior clinician attends.**
2. **Give oxygen if required.**
3. **Obtain IV access/take bloods.**
4. **Give IV antibiotics.**
5. **Give IV fluids.**
6. **Monitor.**

Notes

Levy, M., Evans, L. and Rhodes, A. (2018) *The Surviving Sepsis Campaign Bundle: 2018 Update*. Available at: **bit.ly/SSCB2018**

Sepsis Alliance (2019) *Symptoms*. Available at: **www.sepsis.org/sepsis/symptoms**

7.1 Angina

Angina is a pain or discomfort felt in the chest, which is caused by the heart not receiving an adequate blood (oxygen) supply, resulting in myocardial ischaemia. Angina is caused by the narrowing of the arteries and can present as pain that is sometimes felt in the arm, neck, stomach and jaw.

Types of angina

Stable angina

This is the most common type of angina. It occurs when the heart is working harder than usual; for example, during exercise. The pain usually subsides after a couple of minutes' rest or taking GTN spray (or other angina medications).

Stable angina is not a medical emergency; however, it suggests that a heart attack is more likely to happen.

Unstable angina

Unlike stable angina, unstable angina doesn't follow any pattern. It can occur more often and be more severe. Rest or medication may not relieve the pain.

Unstable angina is very dangerous and requires emergency treatment. Unstable angina could be a sign of an impending myocardial infarction (MI).

Signs and symptoms

Symptoms of angina include:

- chest pain or discomfort, possibly described as pressure, squeezing, burning or fullness
- pain in the arms, neck, jaw, shoulder or back accompanying chest pain
- nausea
- fatigue
- shortness of breath
- sweating
- dizziness.

Treatment

Sublingual GTN is the first-line treatment. It works by causing venous and coronary artery dilation, reducing workload on the heart; this reduces the symptoms experienced by the patient.

If GTN is not effective more medications will be given:

- Oxygen should be given if there is evidence of hypoxia; be wary of CO_2 retainers
- Cannulas to be inserted for IV pain relief
- Aspirin and clopidogrel to be given for antiplatelet effect.

7.2 Myocardial infarction (MI)

Myocardial infarction is defined as the death or necrosis of part of the myocardium due to the reduction or cessation of blood flow. It is commonly known as a heart attack.

MI can either be classified as an ST elevation myocardial infarction (STEMI) or a non-ST elevation myocardial infarction (non-STEMI). STEMI can be seen in a 12-lead ECG where the ST segment is elevated. In a non-STEMI there is no evidence in the ECG, but raised troponin levels in the blood suggest that necrosis has occurred.

Signs and symptoms

- Chest pain – described as a pressure, tightness or squeezing in the centre of the chest
- Radiation of pain to other parts of the body – it can feel as if the pain is travelling from the chest to the arms (usually the left arm is affected, but it can affect both arms), jaw, neck, back and abdomen
- Light-headedness or dizziness
- Sweating
- Shortness of breath
- Nausea or vomiting
- An overwhelming sense of anxiety (similar to having a panic attack)
- Coughing or wheezing.

Assessment

- 12-lead ECG; an important tool for diagnosis (see photo in *Section 14.4*)
- Vital signs
- Blood analysis
- Chest X-ray.

Treatment

The aim of care is to:

- limit the infarction site
- re-establish optimal cardiac output
- relieve pain.

This can be effected by:

- detecting and preventing any life-threatening complications
- reperfusion therapies – PCI (percutaneous coronary intervention) and thrombolytic therapy
- pain relief.

Reassuring the patient is very important here. The person is often aware of the situation and can feel extremely panicked. You can help by talking to them.

> Carefully consider chest pain presentation in women, people with diabetes and the elderly, as they can present differently from the norm. Women are more likely than men to have symptoms such as fatigue, neck pain, syncope, nausea, right arm pain, dizziness and jaw pain.

Shockable and non-shockable rhythms will be discussed in *Chapter 15*.

Notes

A stroke is when the blood supply to part of the brain is interrupted. This results in brain cells receiving less oxygen and nutrients that are essential for brain function. Without blood, brain cells can become damaged and could die.

There are two different types of stroke.

An **ischaemic stroke** occurs when a blood vessel supplying the brain with blood becomes blocked.

A **haemorrhagic stroke** occurs when a blood vessel in the brain ruptures (a bleed on the brain).

A **transient ischaemic attack** (TIA) is sometimes called a mini-stroke. This is caused by a temporary clot that dislodges itself. A TIA can be recognised following the FAST test (see *Section 8.2*) and signs and symptoms will last no longer than 24 hours. A TIA is not a stroke but should be taken seriously as it is a major warning sign for strokes.

8.1 Signs and symptoms of stroke

Signs and symptoms can vary from patient to patient. Not all signs and symptoms need to be present for a stroke to be suspected.

- Weakness in limbs or facial muscles
- Drooping of the face
- Numbness, tingling or loss of sensation in the face or limbs
- Varying levels of consciousness
- Acute memory impairment
- Speech and language difficulties
- Double vision, or loss of vision
- Changes to hearing

- Impaired balance
- Ataxia (not being able to control the movements of the body)
- Nausea, vomiting
- Severe headache.

8.2 Assessment of stroke

1 Remember FAST!

Face – ask the person to smile and watch for a droop, on either side of the face.

Arms – ask the person to lift both arms. Are they symmetrical?

Speech – is the person's speech slurred? Does what they are saying make sense?

Time – if you see any of these symptoms, it's time to alert another professional.

The FAST test has been designed to help identify if someone is suffering from a potential stroke or TIA.

A CT or MRI scan of the head will be used to identify if a stroke has taken place and if so, whether it is an ischaemic or haemorrhagic stroke.

To help determine the type, location and cause of a stroke, physicians may use:

- a CT or MRI scan of the head – to see the type and/or cause of the stroke
- ECG – to see if there are any problems with the heart's conduction system that could have caused the stroke
- carotid ultrasound – to see if there are any narrowing or blockages in the carotid arteries.

If you think someone you are caring for is having a stroke, complete the FAST test and get help immediately.

8.3 Treatment of stroke

A stroke is a medical emergency and should be treated as quickly as possible.

Ischaemic stroke treatment

The aim of treatment is to break apart or dislodge the clot.

Thrombolysis

Thrombolysis is the delivery of a medication called alteplase, or recombinant tissue plasminogen activator (rt-PA). Thrombolysis can break down and disperse a clot that is preventing blood from reaching the brain. Thrombolysis needs to be given within 4½ hours of the onset of stroke symptoms. In some cases, it can be given up to 6 hours after symptoms start; however, the longer the delay before thrombolysis, the less effective the treatment is.

All people with a diagnosis of ischaemic stroke should be given 300 mg of aspirin as soon as possible. A daily dose of 300 mg should be continued for two weeks after the onset of stroke symptoms. Long-term antithrombotic treatment should be started after the two weeks of aspirin.

Haemorrhagic stroke treatment

The aim of treatment is to stop the bleeding. Treatment will involve surgery. A craniectomy (surgical opening of the skull) will be performed to give the surgeon access to clip the aneurysm and stop the bleeding. Alternatively a decompressive hemicraniectomy may be performed; this is a surgical opening of the skull to allow space for the brain to swell.

Notes

American Stroke Association (2019) *Stroke Symptoms*. Available at: www.stroke.org/en/about-stroke/stroke-symptoms

NICE (2019) NG128: *Stroke and Transient Ischaemic Attack in Over 16s: diagnosis and initial management*. Available at: www.nice.org.uk/guidance/ng128

Royal College of Nursing (2019) *Stroke*. Available at: www.rcn.org.uk/clinical-topics/neuroscience-nursing/stroke

A fracture is simply a broken bone. A bone can be fractured in a number of different ways.

A *traumatic* fracture is a fracture that has been caused by trauma. A *pathological* fracture is a fracture that has occurred from repeated strain on the same area of the body.

9.1 Types of fracture

The two main types of fracture are closed and open fractures.

Closed or simple fracture – when there is a clean break through the bone and the bone ends do not protrude through the skin.

Open or compound fracture – when there is a clean break through the bone and part of the bone does protrude out of the skin. This type of fracture can lead to an increase in infection and blood loss.

Hairline fracture – when a bone cracks but does not break apart.

Comminuted fracture – when there are more than two bone fragments in the break.

Greenstick fracture – when the bone bends and cracks but does not break. These fractures occur in children and adolescents as their bones are less brittle and this causes them to bend.

American Academy of Orthopaedic Surgeons (2019) *Fractures (Broken Bones)*. [online] Available at: https://orthoinfo.aaos.org/en/diseases--conditions/fractures-broken-bones (accessed 17 December 2019).

9.2 Signs and symptoms of fracture

- Pain
- Redness
- Swelling
- Stiffness
- Visible deformity
- Bruising.

9.3 Assessment of fracture

In order to identify if a bone has broken, an X-ray should be carried out. This will also give information on the type and location of the fracture.

9.4 Treatment of fracture

Top tip

Be wary of fractures, especially in people who have sustained trauma. The movements of fracture could cause/introduce internal damage, leading to further complications.

Moving a person with a fracture can also be extremely painful and it could cause further damage to the affected area. Be extremely cautious when treating a person with a confirmed or suspected spinal fracture, to avoid further injury.

Bones have their own self-repair mechanism. The self-repair process begins immediately after the fracture occurs and the healing process can take a few weeks to a few months, depending on the type of fracture and health and age of the person.

However, medical interventions can be introduced to assist and speed up the bone healing process:

Closed reduction – the bone fragments are realigned via manipulation and a cast or splint is applied.

Open reduction – metal plates, screws and wires are placed surgically and are used to hold the bones in alignment. A cast or splint may also be applied.

Traction – the bones are held in place through a pulling force. This is used when fractures occur on the long bone and can also help to alleviate pain.

Notes

_____

_____

_____

_____

_____

_____

_____

_____

Toolkit

SBAR is a systematic method of delivering patient information. By following this method professionals are able to hand over all relevant information in an easy to follow manner. This ensures that no significant information is missed and therefore that the patient's safety is not compromised.

Situation	**Concise statement of the problem**
	• I am .... (your name/role/ward)
	• I am calling about patient Y
	• I am concerned that ... (e.g. BP is low/high, pulse is XX, temperature is XX, Early Warning Score is XX)
Background	**Brief information or history related to the situation**
	• Patient Y was admitted on (XX date) with ... (e.g. MI/chest infection)
	• They have had (X operation/procedure/investigation)
	• Their condition has changed in the last (XX mins)
	• Their last set of obs were (XX)
	• Patient's normal condition is ... (e.g. alert/drowsy/confused/pain-free)
Assessment	**Assessment – the reason you are calling, your assessment findings**
	• I think the problem is (XXX)
	• I have ..... (e.g. given O$_2$/analgesia, stopped the infusion)
	OR
	• I am not sure what the problem is, but patient Y is deteriorating
	OR
	• I don't know what's wrong, but I am really worried

Recommendation	**Action required – what you want from the person you are calling**
	• I need you to come to see the patient in the next (XX mins) AND
	• Is there anything I need to do in the meantime?

Many students get nervous at the thought of handing over; however, SBARs are carried out every day by nurses without them even realising.

Example of a conversation between a student nurse and a consultant in ICU

S: Hi, I am Rachel, 3rd year student nurse. I was wondering if you could take a look at Samantha Jones? I am concerned that she is hypotensive.

B: As you know, Mrs Jones was admitted on Wednesday 4th May following an elective Hartmann's procedure. Her BP was stable overnight sitting at around 110/90. However, her BP has been dropping this morning and is currently 90/70. She is normally easily rousable; however, she is now drowsy. She is currently not on any medication to control her BP.

A: I think the problem is that she is hypotensive, and we need to do something quickly to bring her BP back up to normal.

R: I need you to you come quickly and have a look at Mrs Jones and I think she may benefit from an infusion of noradrenaline.

11.1 Understanding ABGs

An arterial blood gas or ABG test measures the acidity, pH and the levels of oxygen and carbon dioxide from an arterial blood sample. This test can be used to check a patient's lung function and how effective the gas exchange is. This test is done at the bedside where blood is taken from the artery and placed into a tube to be sent to be tested.

Interpreting ABG results can be hard to grasp at the start. Before getting stuck into the details of the analysis, it's important to consider the person and their condition, as this provides essential context to the ABG result.

Normal ranges

pH: 7.35–7.45

$PaCO_2$: 4.7–6.0 kPa

PaO_2: 11–13 kPa

HCO_3^-: 22–26 mEq/L

Base excess: −2 to +2 mmol/L

Oxygenation (PaO_2)

Always consider oxygenation first.

- PaO_2 should be >11 kPa on air in a healthy patient.
- This changes if the patient is receiving oxygen therapy. Their PaO_2 should be approximately 10 kPa less than the % inspired concentration (so a patient on 30% oxygen would be expected to have a PaO_2 of approximately 20 kPa).

Hypoxaemia

If the PaO_2 is <10 kPa on air – the patient is hypoxaemic. Hypoxia represents an abnormally low oxygen content in any tissue or organ, or the body as a whole.

If the PaO_2 is <8 kPa on air – the patient is severely hypoxaemic and in respiratory failure.

pH

The body has a narrow range for pH of the body and small abnormalities in pH have very significant and wide-ranging effects on the physiology of the human body. Therefore, it is essential to pay close attention to pH abnormalities.

1 **Is the pH normal, acidotic or alkalotic?**

- Acidotic: pH <7.35
- Normal: pH 7.35–7.45
- Alkalotic: pH >7.45

Once you've worked out if it is acidic or alkalotic, you need to think about what has caused the change in pH. The cause can either be metabolic or respiratory. The changes in pH are caused by an imbalance in the CO_2 (respiratory) or HCO_3^- (metabolic).

$PaCO_2$

Before looking at CO_2, you know the pH and the PaO_2. So, for example, you have identified that your patient's pH is abnormal but you don't yet know the cause. There are two options that can cause abnormalities in pH:

- It could be respiratory (abnormal level of CO_2)
- It could be metabolic (abnormal level of HCO_3^- (bicarbonate) which is a by-product of the body's metabolism).

The level of CO_2 quickly helps rule in or out the respiratory system as the cause for the abnormal pH.

	pH	CO_2	HCO_3^-
Respiratory acidosis	↓	↑	Normal
Respiratory alkalosis	↑	↓	Normal
Respiratory acidosis with metabolic compensation	↓/↔	↑	↑
Respiratory alkalosis with metabolic compensation	↑/↔	↓	↓

HCO_3^-

HCO_3^- is a base, which helps remove acids (H^+ ions). So when HCO_3^- is raised, the pH is increased as there are fewer free H^+ ions, causing alkalosis. When HCO_3^- is low, the pH is decreased as there are more free H^+ ions, causing acidosis.

	pH	HCO_3^-	CO_2
Metabolic acidosis	↓	↓	Normal
Metabolic alkalosis	↑	↑	Normal
Metabolic acidosis with respiratory compensation	↓	↓	↓
Metabolic alkalosis with respiratory compensation	↑	↑	↑

 Notes

_____

_____

_____

12.1 GCS

The Glasgow Coma Scale (GCS) is used to evaluate response ability. It is commonly used following head injury and as part of neurological observations. GCS observations can be found on the NEWS 2 chart shown on the inside front cover of this book.

There are three categories to the GCS that you are assessing. They are eyes, verbal responses and motor responses. For each section you give a score and then you add them up to get the final score. The maximum score is 15 and the minimum is 3. A healthy person with a normal GCS would score 15.

A paediatric version of the GCS is also available at **bit.ly/P-GCS**

Eyes (max. score of 4 in this section)

1. *No response* – no matter what you do, the person's eyes won't open
2. *To pain* – eyes open to pain
3. *To voice* – eyes open to speech
4. *Open* – eyes open spontaneously

Verbal response (max. score of 5 in this section)

1. *No response* – they are not talking at all
2. *Moans, unintelligible* – they are just making sounds
3. *Nonsensical speech* – they are saying words, but they don't make sense
4. *Disoriented* – they are talking, but are confused
5. *Oriented and alert* – they are talking normally

Motor response (max. score of 6 in this section)

1. *No response* – no matter what you do, the person isn't moving
2. *Decerebrate extension* – if pain is applied, their body flexes away from their core
3. *Decorticate flexion* – if pain is applied, their body tightens towards their core
4. *Withdraws to pain* – if pain is applied, their body tries to back away from the pain spot
5. *Localises pain* – if pain is applied, they move their hand to the pain spot
6. *Follows commands* – they are moving on their own and can obey a two-part command

12.2 Pupil observations

This is done by shining a light into the person's eyes and observing the change in the pupil. The pupil should constrict when the light is shone into it and should dilate once the light has been removed. When shining the light, observe the reactions of both pupils and score them on the NEWS 2 chart.

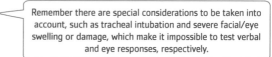

Remember there are special considerations to be taken into account, such as tracheal intubation and severe facial/eye swelling or damage, which make it impossible to test verbal and eye responses, respectively.

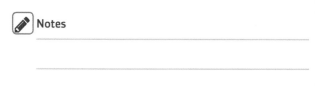

Notes

Observations

Remember when documenting to detail what the person scored for each section. For example:

At 16:00 Sam scored a GCS of 13.

E   3

V   4

M   6

Both pupils were size 3 and equal and reactive. Normal power in all limbs.

Notes

_____

_____

_____

_____

_____

_____

_____

_____

_____

_____

The analysis of urine can provide us with important information about a patient's health which can assist in the diagnosis of medical conditions. It can also help us monitor the progression of disease and effects of treatment.

13.1 Methods of collecting urine

- Natural voiding into a specimen pot.
- Transfer of urine from bedpan/urinal into a specimen pot.
- Midstream urinalysis (MSU) – genitals must be cleaned to reduce presence of contaminants such as bacteria. Ask the patient to pass urine into the toilet and then catch the middle part of the flow of urine into a sterile container and then pass the remaining urine into the toilet.
- A pad – some clinical areas have kits to enable a urine sample to be collected from an incontinence pad when a patient is unable to follow the above collection methods. The process involves placing a small sterile pad into a clean continence pad. Once the patient has urinated, the pad can be squeezed and a syringe can assist in aspirating the sample. The kit has detailed instructions for use, including the maximum duration that the testing pad can be left in place.
- Catheter specimen of urine (CSU) – clean sampling port of catheter with alcohol-based swab and allow it to dry for 30 seconds. If using a needle-less system, insert syringe into port and aspirate urine (approximately 10 ml). Some ports may require a needle and syringe. Insert needle into port at 45° angle, aspirate and remove needle. Sometimes there isn't enough urine in the catheter tubing to extract, so you may have to clamp the tubing to allow enough urine to accumulate for collection. Remember to unclamp the tubing afterwards to allow drainage to continue.

- Suprapubic aspirate (SPA) – a doctor or advanced nurse practitioner will collect a sterile sample of urine by inserting a needle into the patient's bladder just above the pubic bone.
- 24-hour urine collection – used to assess kidney function by collecting and assessing urine collected over a 24-hour period.

13.2 Physical appearance

Before using a dipstick (reagent) test to analyse urine, consider the colour, clarity and smell of the sample.

Notes

Colour	
Light yellow or straw colour	Normal
Dark yellow	May indicate patient is dehydrated
Bright red or reddish-brown	May suggest blood in the urine (haematuria)
Brown–green or strong yellow	May suggest bilirubin is present, which can be indicative of liver or gall bladder problems
Clarity	
Clear	Normal
Cloudy or containing small particles of debris	May be due to presence of pus, protein or white blood cells, which can be indicative of infection, kidney stones or urinary stasis
Smell	
Very little smell	Normal
'Fishy' smell	May indicate presence of infection, or that a sample has been waiting too long to be tested – a sample should be tested within 2 hours of collection
Sweet or fruity smell	May suggest presence of ketone bodies which are by-products of fat metabolism and may indicate patients who have been fasting or have diabetic hyperglycaemia (see table in *Section 13.3*)

i Top tip

Some foods and medications can produce certain smells (e.g. asparagus) or can alter the colour of urine (e.g. beetroot).

13.3 Urine analysis

Reagent strips are a quick, easy and non-invasive way of testing urine. It is important that you understand what the findings mean so that you can report any abnormalities to your practice supervisor – see below.

Test	Normal value	Common cause of change
Leucocytes	Not usually found in urine	The presence of leucocytes is an indication of a renal/bladder urinary tract infection (UTI)
Nitrates	Not usually found in urine	Presence suggests a UTI
Protein	Normal urine has low levels of the proteins albumin and globulin which are not enough to give a positive reagent strip reaction	High levels may suggest UTI, renal conditions, heart failure, pre-eclampsia
pH	4.5–8.0	Low pH (strongly acidic, pH <4) may be caused by diabetes, starvation and dehydration High pH (alkaline, pH >8) may indicate stale urine which is unsuitable for further testing
Blood (haematuria)	Not usually found in urine	Haematuria may suggest renal or urinary tract conditions

Look out for a false positive if a female is menstruating

Test	Normal value	Common cause of change
Specific gravity Tests the concentration and diluting abilities of the kidneys	1.005–1.030	High concentration may indicate dehydration

Low concentration indicates very dilute urine which may be because of a high fluid intake or may be caused by renal abnormalities |
| **Ketones** Ketones are produced by the breakdown of fatty acid | Not usually found in urine | These may be present because of fasting (e.g. vomiting) or uncontrolled diabetes |
| **Glucose** | Not usually found in urine | Presence may be associated with raised blood glucose (diabetes), pregnancy and renal abnormalities |

i Tips for urinalysis

- Before you begin urinalysis, check the expiry date of the reagent strips and make sure that the container hasn't been left open.
- Wash your hands before and after – always wear gloves.
- Use a fresh urine sample to ensure the best results.
- When removing the strip from the urine sample, run the edges of the strip against the container or a paper towel to remove excess urine.
- Hold reagent strip close to the colour blocks on the bottle of the reagent strips to match carefully.
- Wait for the time recommended by the urinalysis reagent strips, to ensure accurate results.
- Record the results and report any abnormalities to your practice supervisor or a staff nurse.

4   ECG types, diagram and reading a rhythm strip

An electrocardiogram (ECG) records the direction and size of the electrical current caused by the depolarisation and repolarisation of the heart.

There are many different types of ECG. This chapter will detail why different ECGs are used, how to read ECGs and how to correctly place the leads.

A 3-lead, 5-lead or 12-lead ECG can be used. The more leads that are placed, the more areas of the heart that can be observed.

14.1 Why use cardiac monitoring?

A patient may require cardiac monitoring for a number of reasons, including:

- chest pain
- shock
- major trauma
- following major surgery
- palpitations
- post cardiac/respiratory arrest.

No matter the type of ECG, the steps taken to place the ECG are still the same

1. Gain consent from the patient.
2. Ensure that the patient's privacy is upheld as much as possible; close the curtains and remove anyone who does not need to be in the room.
3. If the skin is oily or sweaty, dry it. If the patient's body hair is particularly long where the electrodes are going to be attached, you may need to trim it.

14.2 3-lead ECG

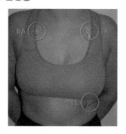

RA – red	Electrode placed under right clavicle near right shoulder within the ribcage frame
LA – yellow	Electrode placed under left clavicle near left shoulder within the ribcage frame
LL – green	Electrode placed on the left side below pectoral muscles at lower edge of left ribcage

14.3 5-lead ECG

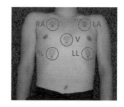

RA – red	Electrode placed under right clavicle near right shoulder within the ribcage frame
LA – yellow	Electrode placed under left clavicle near left shoulder within the ribcage frame
LL – green	Electrode placed on the left side below pectoral muscles at lower edge of left ribcage

V – white	Electrode placed on the fourth intercostal space at right sternal border
RL – black	Electrode placed on a non-muscular surface on the lower edge of the right ribcage

14.4 12-lead ECG

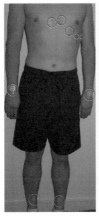 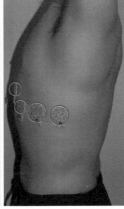

Top tip

Remember that with ECGs leads, it's the number of views you are seeing of the heart, and not the number of electrodes placed, that is relevant.

You are placing 10 electrodes but are able to see 12 different areas of the heart – hence the term '12-lead ECG'.

Chest leads

V1 – red (C1)	Fourth intercostal space at the right sternal edge

V2 – yellow (C2)	Fourth intercostal space at the left sternal edge
V3 – green (C3)	Midway between V2 and V4
V4 – brown (C4)	Fifth intercostal space in the midclavicular line
V5 – black (C5)	Left anterior axillary line at the same horizontal level as V4
V6 – purple (C6)	Left mid-axillary line at the same horizontal level as V4 and V5

Limb leads

Right arm lead (RAL)	Right forearm, proximal to wrist left arm lead
Left arm lead (LAL)	Left forearm, proximal to wrist right arm lead
Left leg lead (LL)	Left lower leg, proximal to ankle right leg lead
Right leg lead (RL)	Right lower leg, proximal to ankle left leg lead

14.5 Reading a rhythm strip

Being able to understand and interpret ECG readings is a very complex skill and can take a long time to master. Do not expect to learn this skill as quickly as you learn other skills. Before you attempt to interpret an ECG, refresh yourself on the PQRST complex.

Campbell, B., Richley, D., Ross, C. and Eggett, C.J. (2017) *Clinical Guidelines by Consensus: recording a standard 12-lead electrocardiogram.* An approved method by the Society for Cardiological Science and Technology (SCST). Available at: www.scst.org.uk/resources/SCST_ECG_Recording_Guidelines_20171.pdf (accessed 17 December 2019)

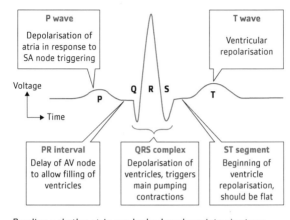

P wave	T wave
Depolarisation of atria in response to SA node triggering	Ventricular repolarisation

Voltage

Time

P Q R S T

PR interval	QRS complex	ST segment
Delay of AV node to allow filling of ventricles	Depolarisation of ventricles, triggers main pumping contractions	Beginning of ventricle repolarisation, should be flat

Reading a rhythm strip can be broken down into six steps.

Step 1   Is there any electrical activity?

If there is no electrical activity a flat line will appear on the screen. Seek help immediately and begin CPR. The patient's heart has stopped beating and will need to be resuscitated.

If there is electrical activity continue to the next step.

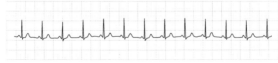

Rhythm strip with electrical activity.

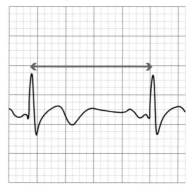

Rhythm strip with no electrical activity.

> Step 2   What is the ventricular QRS rate?

The QRS rate is the heart rate.

This is calculated by counting the big boxes between the top R waves and dividing this number into 300.

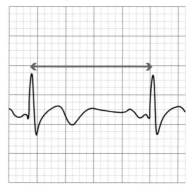

There are roughly four big boxes.

$$\frac{300}{4} = 75 \text{ beats per minute (bpm)}$$

Step 3   Is the QRS rate regular or irregular?

This shows us whether the heart is beating regularly or
irregularly. To determine if the rate is regular or irregular take
a sheet of paper and line it up parallel with the rhythm strip.
Mark on the paper with a pen where the R waves are and
move this along the strip. If the pen marks correlate with the
other R waves along the strip, then the heart is beating
regularly.

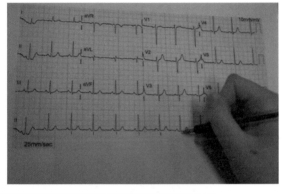

Step 4   Is the QRS complex width normal or prolonged?

A normal QRS complex should be narrowed and no longer
than three small boxes. If QRS complex is normal this shows
atrial activity.

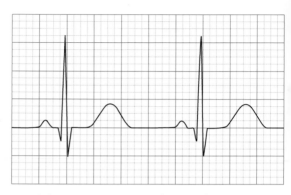

Normal QRS, as no longer than 3 small boxes (atrial activity).

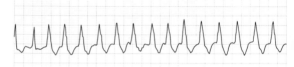

Prolonged QRS, as longer than 3 boxes (ventricular activity).

Step 5   Is there atrial activity present?

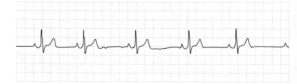

If a P wave is present, there is atrial activity.

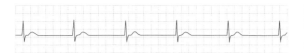

If there is no P wave present, this shows ventricular activity.

Step 6   How is the atrial activity related to ventricular activity?

For every P wave a QRS complex should follow. If there is not, something is abnormal and the ECG should be brought to the doctor's attention.

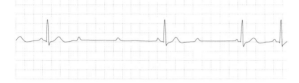

QRS complex does not follow after every P wave.

Shockable and non-shockable rhythms will be discussed in *Chapter 15*.

14.6 Worked example

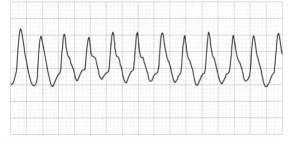

1. Is there electrical activity?
2. What is the QRS rate?
3. Is the QRS rate regular or irregular?
4. Is the QRS complex width normal or prolonged?
5. Is atrial activity present?
6. How is atrial activity related to ventricular activity?

Answers to worked example

1. Yes
2. 300/1.5 = 200 bpm (tachycardic)
3. Regular
4. Prolonged as there are more than three small boxes (ventricular activity)
5. Yes, as the P wave is present
6. There is no P wave for every QRS complex, and so there is no relation

This is ventricular tachycardia.

Notes

Shockable and non-shockable rhythms

5

A shockable rhythm is a rhythm caused by an aberration in the electrical conduction of the heart. Defibrillation can be used to 'reset' the heart to its normal rhythm. Rhythms that are not responsive to shock are pulseless electrical activity (PEA) and asystole. In these cases, identifying and reversing the primary cause, CPR and administering adrenaline are the only tools you have to resuscitate the patient.

15.1 Shockable rhythms

A defibrillator should be used to shock patients into a safer rhythm (see *Section 3.4* for placement of defib pads). The shock restarts the heart's electrical conduction system. Call for help immediately if you need to use a defibrillator.

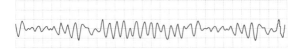

Ventricular fibrillation (VF).

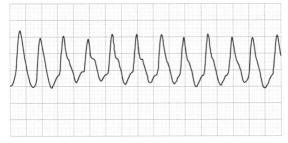

Ventricular tachycardia (VT).

15.2 Non-shockable rhythms

Not every rhythm is shockable. In cases where the rhythm is non-shockable and the patient has arrested, the management plan should be to treat the cause of the arrest (4 Hs and 4 Ts, see *Section 3.5*).

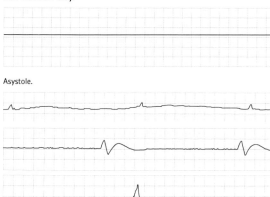

Asystole.

Pulseless electrical activity (PEA).

📝 Notes

People who are in an acute care setting will most likely be experiencing some form of pain. It is important to remember that those who are unconscious can also experience pain. As nurses our role includes observing for signs that someone is pain.

16.1 Assessment of pain

Pain can be assessed whether the patient is conscious or unconscious.

If the patient is unconscious

The FLACC behavioural scale, shown below, can be used in such patients. This scale was developed to assess pain in young children but it can also be used in adults who are unable to communicate.

- Observe for at least 5 minutes.
- Observe body and legs uncovered.
- If possible, reposition the patient.
- Touch the body and assess for tenseness and tone.

Each category is scored from 0–2 which results in a total score of 0–10.

✎ Notes

_____

_____

_____

_____

FLACC Scale – Pain Assessment Tool

	Date/Time						
Face 0 – No particular expression or smile 1 – Occasional grimace or frown, withdrawn, disinterested 2 – Frequent to constant quivering chin, clenched jaw							
Legs 0 – Normal position or relaxed 1 – Uneasy, restless, tense 2 – Kicking, or legs drawn up							
Activity 0 – Lying quietly, normal position, moves easily 1 – Squirming, shifting back and forth, tense 2 – Arched, rigid or jerking							
Cry 0 – No cry (awake or asleep) 1 – Moans or whimpers; occasional complaint 2 – Crying steadily, screams or sobs, frequent complaints							
Consolability 0 – Content, relaxed 1 – Reassured by occasional touching, hugging or being talked to, distractible 2 – Difficult to console or comfort							
Total Score							

0 = Relaxed and comfortable

1–3 = Mild discomfort

4–6 = Moderate pain

7–10 = Severe discomfort/pain

An accurate measure of pain can help the medical team to determine the appropriate pain management treatment.

If the patient is conscious

Ask the patient to score their pain on a scale from 0 (no pain at all) to 10 (the worst pain imaginable). The ladder tool shown below can be used to assist with this: ask your patients to point to the face that best represents their pain. This system works particularly well with children, people with neurological impairments as well as people with learning disabilities and dementia.

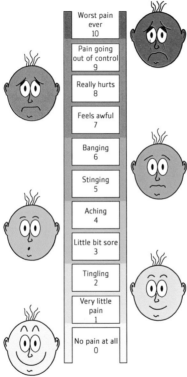

Ladder tool for describing pain.

Alternatively, use the FLACC scale:

- Observe for at least 2–5 minutes.
- Observe legs and body uncovered.
- Reposition patient or observe activity; assess body for tenseness and tone.
- Initiate consoling interventions if needed.

16.2 Managing pain

Once a patient's pain has been assessed, we must manage their pain. There are two approaches to pain management – pharmacological management and non-pharmacological management.

Managing pain pharmacologically refers to the use of drugs such as paracetamol, ibuprofen, codeine, morphine and other analgesic medication.

Non-pharmacological management of pain refers to interventions that do not involve medication. Massage, distraction or mindfulness are just a few of the methods which can be used to treat pain without the use of medication.

In critical care areas you are more likely to see pharmacological intervention. However, combining the use of medication and non-pharmacological methods can help to treat your patients' pain better.

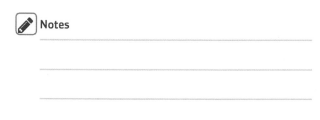 **Notes**

Medication should not be prescribed by trade name; rather it should always be in the generic form.

Reason for medication (commonly referred to as)	Medication group	Medication name (not an exhaustive list)
Pain relief	Analgesics	Paracetamol, ibuprofen, co-codamol, codeine, tramadol and morphine sulphate
Nausea	Anti-emetic	Metoclopramide, ondansetron, promethazine hydrochloride, cyclizine
Cholesterol-reducing	Statins	Atorvastatin, simvastatin, lovastatin
Blood thinner	Antiplatelet drugs, anticoagulants	Rivaroxaban, aspirin, heparin, warfarin
Water pill	Diuretic	Furosemide, bendroflumethiazide
Itch/allergy	Antipruritic	Antihistamines (diphenhydramine), corticosteroids (topical (e.g. betamethasone) and oral (e.g. prednisone))
Lowers blood pressure	Antihypertensive	Calcium channel blockers (amlodipine), ACE inhibitors (lisinopril, ramipril), beta-blockers (atenolol, metoprolol)
Bacterial infection	Antibiotics	Penicillins (amoxicillin), erythromycin, clarithromycin, azithromycin, ciprofloxacin, levofloxacin, vancomycin, metronidazole

Constipation	Laxatives	Docusate, senna, suppositories, polyethylene glycol, milk of magnesia
Irregular heartbeat	Anti-arrhythmics	Digoxin

✎ Notes

_____

_____

_____

_____

_____

_____

_____

_____

_____

_____

_____

_____

Difficult conversations

On our placements we were involved with many conversations that involved delivering "bad news". What "bad news" is varies from person to person. For one person a cancer diagnosis may be bad news while for another, bad news might be that they need to wait three hours for pharmacy to get their prescription ready.

We have included a section on difficult conversations to give students guidance and reassurance on how to care for people when bad news has been broken.

There is no step by step guide for having difficult conversations. It is important to remember that each difficult conversation you have will be different. This is because you are speaking to individuals and families with different life experiences, beliefs and values, expectations, relationships, understanding and emotions.

The following are tips based on our own experiences.

Be honest

If you are asked a difficult question by a patient or family member and you don't know the answer, be honest and tell the individual that you are unsure of the answer. Tell them that although you don't know, you will go and find out the answer for them, or ask someone more experienced to answer their questions.

Listen to the person

Listening to someone's concerns and worries can be hugely beneficial to them. It may not feel that you are doing much by listening, but you are giving the person an opportunity to voice their thoughts and feelings.

What does the person understand?

After any news has been broken, it can be difficult for someone to remember all the information they have been given. Many people are often anxious about what they don't know. It is important to take the time to go over what the patient understands about their situation so that you can help fill in any gaps, make it clearer and help to relieve some of the anxiety. It can also be beneficial for some people to have the information written down so that they can read it when they need to. Encourage them to write down further questions as they think of them.

Be aware of your own emotions and needs

Students can be put in situations that are upsetting and hard to deal with. If you experience any conversations or emotions that are difficult to deal with, speak to your practice supervisor and let them know how you are feeling. It is important we look after ourselves so that we can look after our patients. Reflection, and the ability to recognise the need to seek support to make sense of situations, are key professional skills.

Notes

_____

_____

_____

_____

_____

One of the best sources of advice for students is undoubtedly other students. We recognise that the hints and tips we have been given during our learning are some of the most valuable resources we have, and we share these with you here.

- Critical care areas can be intimidating; however, it's important to remain calm and remember that in these areas there is more support for students.
- Focus on the person first – it can be easy to become overwhelmed by the technology and machines but always concentrate on the person first.
- Seek out opportunities – if the arrest/airway trolley is being used, get involved and ask to observe things you haven't seen before.
- Carry a notebook or jot things in the *Notes* spaces in this book – you won't remember everything you get told all day so write it down and look it up later.
- Do some research about your area – you won't be expected to know it all but researching general topics in your area is a good idea and gives you a bit of confidence.
- Have confidence in yourself – this is a new area, but you already have a wealth of knowledge and skills. Your core nursing skills are just as valuable in these areas.
- Work within your ability and have the confidence to say that you don't feel confident doing something.
- Ask lots of questions – everyone has experience and knowledge for you to learn from.
- It is OK to take some time out if it gets too much. Speak up and talk with your practice supervisor or your peers. Everyone needs support.
- Breathe – stay calm.

Notes

Resources

The table below shows normal vital sign ranges and blood glucose parameters (adults).

Respiratory rate	12–20 breaths per minute
Pulse rate	60–100 beats per minute
Blood pressure range	100/60 – 140/80 mmHg
Blood glucose	4–7 mmol/L

The following table gives metric units and their equivalents.

Unit	Abbreviation	Equivalent	Abbreviation
1 kilogram	kg	1000 grams	g
1 gram	g	1000 milligrams	mg
1 milligram	mg	1000 micrograms	mcg*
1 microgram	mcg	1000 nanograms	ng*
1 litre	L or l	1000 millilitres	ml
1 mole	mol	1000 millimoles	mmol
1 millimole	mmol	1000 micromoles	mcmol

*It is recommended that micrograms and nanograms should never be abbreviated

American Stroke Association (2019) *Types of Stroke*. Available at: www.strokeassociation.org/en/about-stroke/types-of-stroke (accessed 17 December 2019)

British Heart Foundation (2019) *What is an electrocardiogram (ECG)?* Heart Matters. Available at: www.bhf.org.uk/informationsupport/heart-matters-magazine/medical/tests/electrocardiogram-ecg (accessed 17 December 2019)

Chest Heart & Stroke Scotland (2019) *What is a Stroke?* Available at: www.chss.org.uk/stroke-information-and-support/strokes-and-tias-transient-ischaemic-attack/what-is-a-stroke (accessed 17 December 2019)

Coventry, L., Finn, J. and Bremner, A. (2011) Sex differences in symptom presentation in acute myocardial infarction: a systematic review and meta-analysis. *Heart & Lung*, **40**(6): 477–491.

Kaufman, D.A. (2019) *Interpretation of ABGs*. American Thoracic Society. Available at: www.thoracic.org/professionals/clinical-resources/critical-care/clinical-education/abgs.php (accessed 17 December 2019)

Kleinpell, R.M., Schorr, C.A. and Balk, R.A. (2016) The new sepsis definitions: implications for critical care practitioners. *American Journal of Critical Care*, **25**(5): 457–464. Available at: ajcc.aacnjournals.org/content/25/5/457.full (accessed 17 December 2019)

Practical Clinical Skills (2019) *Sinus Tachycardia*. Available at: www.practicalclinicalskills.com/sinus-tachycardia (accessed 17 December 2019)

Radiological Society of North America (2019) *Stroke*. Available at: www.radiologyinfo.org/en/info.cfm?pg=stroke#disease-evaluation (accessed 17 December 2019)

Rawshani, A. (2019) *ECG Interpretation: characteristics of the normal ECG*. Available at: https://ecgwaves.com/ecg-normal-p-wave-qrs-complex-st-segment-t-wave-j-point (accessed 17 December 2019)

Resuscitation Council (2015) *Adult Advanced Life Support*. Available at: www.resus.org.uk/resuscitation-guidelines/adult-advanced-life-support (accessed 17 December 2019)

Roberts, S.J. and Ke, H.Z. (2018) Anabolic strategies to augment bone fracture healing. *Current Osteoporosis Reports*, **16**(3): 289–298. Available at: www.ncbi.nlm.nih.gov/pmc/articles/PMC5945805 (accessed 17 December 2019)

St John Ambulance (2019) Using a Defibrillator (AED). (video). Available at: www.sja.org.uk/sja/first-aid-advice/first-aid-techniques/using-a--defibrillator-aed.aspx (accessed 17 December 2019)

Stroke Association (2019) *Treatments*. Available at: www.stroke.org.uk/what-is-stroke/diagnosis-to-discharge/treatment (accessed 17 December 2019)

The UK Sepsis Trust (2019) *ED/AMU Sepsis Screening & Action Tool*. Available at: https://sepsistrust.org/wp-content/uploads/2018/06/ED-adult-NICE-Final-1107.pdf (accessed 17 December 2019)

Websites

Hearte: Heart Education Awareness Resource and Training Through E-learning

If you are unsure about anything heart related or want to increase your knowledge, this is a great resource. The site can take you through complete modules or you can look for specific information. We found this site particularly helpful for revising ECG lead placement. www.heartelearning.org

National Institute for Health and Care Excellence (NICE) Guidelines

The NICE guidelines are what many hospitals base their current practice criteria on. NICE gives recommendations on a wide array of subjects including medication and medical management of conditions. The guidelines are reviewed regularly to ensure that they are providing the most up-to-date and relevant information.

The NICE guidelines are a great resource to consult if you are unsure on what best practice is, and will always make for a great reference for your essays. www.nice.org.uk

Practical Clinical Skills

This website covers a wide range of practical skills. It is designed for students to use and contains many interactive elements. There are a number of detailed explanations and lots of quizzes to test yourself. If you learn better by doing than reading, you'll definitely want to visit this website. www.practicalclinicalskills.com

Resuscitation Council (UK)

This is a fantastic website for all things related to resuscitation. It gives more specific information on drugs used during resuscitation and the quality standards that the NHS abides by. It is a very student-friendly website and it is reviewed regularly to ensure the most up-to-date and relevant information is given. www.resus.org.uk

Stroke Association/Chest Heart & Stroke Scotland

If you are interested in reading more about strokes, the Stroke Association is a good place to start. The website is designed for patients rather than students, so it would not perhaps make the best of references for academic work. However, it gives a good general overview of strokes and also contains patients' own stories which can provide an insight into some of the more holistic needs of your patients. www.stroke.org.uk

Chest Heart & Stroke Scotland provides similar information to that of the Stroke Association. Again, it is designed for patient use but does provide more in-depth information on the treatment of strokes. CHSS also provides great explanations of angina and MIs. www.chss.org.uk

The UK Sepsis Trust/Sepsis Alliance

These two organisations both provide excellent information on sepsis. The explanations go into more physiological details in all aspects of sepsis and so could be used in academic work. If you are looking to really understand sepsis, we would highly recommend taking the time to look over both of these websites. https://sepsistrust.org and www.sepsis.org

Notes

Notes

Notes